I0703351

MAKEUP FOR BEGINNERS

The ultimate guide to Unleashing
Your Inner Beauty, By Unlocking
the Secrets of Flawless Makeup,
for enthusiastic Beginners

Leonard Lincoln

Table of Contents

CHAPTER ONE

Introduction to Makeup

Makeup is a method of self-expression and enhancement that has been used for generations to improve appearance and create unique looks. It encompasses a wide range of materials and techniques intended to enhance face features, fix flaws, and produce various effects. Makeup, from everyday natural appearances to spectacular evening styles, can be an effective tool for boosting confidence and expressing uniqueness.

Makeup goods include foundations, concealers, powders, eyeshadows, eyeliners, mascaras, lipsticks, and more. Each product is intended to serve a specific goal, such as balancing skin tone, defining eyes, or adding color to lips.

Applying makeup requires a series of processes, beginning with skincare to produce a smooth canvas. This is followed by the application of foundation to balance out skin tone, concealer to conceal blemishes and dark circles, and powder to set the makeup and minimize shine.

Eye makeup normally consists of eyeshadow to add color and depth, eyeliner to define the eyes, and mascara to lengthen and volumize the lashes. Lip makeup entails using lipstick or lip gloss to impart color and sparkle to the lips.

Blending is an important technique in makeup application to provide a smooth and natural appearance. It entails delicately mixing various colors and textures together to eliminate harsh lines and provide a harmonious image.

Makeup can be used to achieve a variety of looks, including subtle and natural to bold and dramatic. It's a diverse art form that allows people to express themselves creatively while also enhancing their characteristics, making them feel confident and beautiful.

Makeup Tools and Product

Foundation evens out skin tone and provides a smooth background for other makeup. It comes in a variety of forms, including as liquid, cream, powder, and stick. For a more natural effect, use a hue that matches your skin tone and undertone.

Concealer is used to hide blemishes, dark circles, and other defects. It is available in a variety of formulas to address specific concerns, such as liquid for under-eye circles and creamy for blemishes. Choose a tint that is similar to your skin tone or slightly lighter for highlighting.

Powder sets foundation and concealer, mattifies the skin, and blurs flaws. It comes in either pressed or loose form. Select a tint that complements your skin tone or is translucent for a natural look.

Brushes: Makeup brushes come in a variety of forms and sizes to suit different needs. Some typical categories are:

Foundation Brush: Used to apply liquid or cream foundation with a flawless finish.

Concealer Brush: A little brush used for applying and blending concealer properly.

Powder Brush: A large, fluffy brush used to distribute setting powder evenly.

Blush Brush: A soft, angled brush used for applying blush to the cheeks.

Eyeshadow Brush: A small, dense brush used for applying eyeshadow to the eyelids.

Eyeliner Brush: A thin, angled brush used for applying eyeliner to the lash line.

Lip Brush: A small, precise brush for applying lipstick or lip gloss.

Tips for Selecting the Right Makeup

Foundation: Test foundation colors on your jawline or neck in natural light to determine the best match for your skin tone. Consider your skin type (dry, oily, or combo) when selecting a formulation (for example, matte for oily skin, moisturizing for dry skin).

Concealer: To ensure flawless blending, use a concealer shade that complements your foundation. Choose a creamy formula for dry skin or a matte texture for oily skin. For highlighting, choose a tint that is lighter than your skin tone.

Powder: Choose a powder hue that complements your skin tone or is translucent for a natural look.

Use a gentle touch to avoid a cakey appearance.

Brushes: Choose brushes that are appropriate for the makeup items you use and the application style you want. Consider the brush's size, shape, and material for best results.

Skin Tone: Use your skin tone (warm, cool, neutral) and undertone (pink, yellow, olive) to choose makeup tones that match your complexion. Warm undertones complement shades with yellow or peach overtones, whilst cool undertones complement shades with pink or blue undertones.

Experiment with various products and tools to determine what works best for you, and don't be hesitant

to seek guidance from makeup
artists or beauty consultants

CHAPTER TWO

Applying foundation for a natural look

Preparing Your Skin: Begin with clean, moisturized skin. If desired, use a primer to create a smoother makeup application with longer-lasting results.

Choose the Right Foundation: Choose a foundation that complements your skin tone and type. Apply a tiny quantity of foundation to the center of your face with a damp makeup sponge or foundation brush, then blend outwards for a smooth finish.

Blend Well: Apply the foundation to your skin with gentle patting motions. Pay special attention to regions that may require additional coverage, such as around the nose and mouth.

Build Coverage as Needed: If you require more coverage, apply a second layer of foundation to the areas that require it, following the same blending technique.

Set with Powder: Use a translucent setting powder to help your foundation last longer and decrease shine. Using a fluffy brush, apply a thin layer of powder over your entire face, focusing on oily areas.

Concealing blemishes and dark circles

Choose the Right Concealer: Choose a concealer that is the same or slightly lighter as your skin tone. For imperfections, use a concealer that complements your foundation. To neutralize dark circles, use a concealer with a peach or orange undertone.

Use a small brush or your fingers to apply concealer directly on blemishes or dark circles. To get a smooth finish, gently blend the edges using a makeup sponge or brush.

Set with Powder: Use a translucent setting powder to keep your concealer from creasing and to guarantee long-lasting coverage.

For a long-lasting finish, set your makeup with powder

Choose the Right Powder: Use a translucent setting powder that matches your skin tone. If you want a matte finish, avoid powders that include shimmer.

Apply Powder: Using a fluffy brush, apply a thin layer of powder to your entire face, emphasizing on oily areas or areas where you've applied concealer.

Blend Well: To avoid a cakey appearance, blend the powder into your skin with light, sweeping motions.

Highlighting and contouring for Added Dimension

Choose the Right Products: Choose a highlighter that suits your skin tone, as well as a contour powder or cream that is a few shades darker.

Use a small brush or your fingertips to apply highlighter to the high points of your face, such as the tops of your cheekbones, bridge of your nose, and cupid's bow.

Apply Contour: Using a contour brush or an angled brush, apply contour powder or cream to the hollows of your cheeks, the jawline, and the sides of your nose. Blend well for a natural appearance.

Blend Well: For a smooth finish, blend the highlighter and contour into your skin with light, sweeping motions.

Set with Powder: Apply a small dusting of translucent setting powder to your highlighted areas to make the products last longer.

To produce a natural-looking finish, mix well and apply with a light hand. Practice and experimentation can help you discover the techniques and products that best suit your skin type and desired appearance.

Introduction to eyeshadow, eyeliner, and mascara.

Here's an overview of eyeshadow, eyeliner, and mascara, as well as suggestions for selecting eyeshadow colors based on your eye shape, applying eyeliner for different styles, and volumizing and lengthening lashes with mascara

Eyeshadow:

Eyeshadow is used to provide depth and character to the eyes, shape them, and complete your cosmetic appearance.

Eyeshadows come in a variety of textures, including powder, cream, and liquid. Powders are the most common, with a diverse spectrum of colors and finishes.

Use an eyeshadow brush to apply makeup on your eyelids. Begin with a base shade that matches your skin tone, then add darker tones to the crease and outer corners for depth. To highlight, apply lighter hues to the inner corners and brow bones.

Eyeliner:

The purpose of eyeliner is to define and shape the eyes. It can provide a variety of looks, from subtle to spectacular.

There are four types of eyeliners: pencil, gel, liquid, and pens. Pencils are versatile and easy to use, although gels and liquids provide greater precision and longer wear.

Apply eyeliner down the lash line, beginning at the inner corner and going outward. To create a winged effect, stretch the line slightly past the outside corner and flick it upward.

Mascara:

Mascara lengthens, volumizes, and defines the lashes.

Mascara comes in formulas for lengthening, volumizing, curling, and waterproof use. Select a formula based on the desired impact.

Application: Begin at the base of the lashes and wiggle the wand upward to coat each one. Apply additional applications, focusing on the lashes' roots, to add volume.

CHAPTER THREE

Choosing Eyeshadow Colors Based on Your Eye Shape

Hooded Eyes: Use matte hues to contour the crease and provide depth. Avoid glittery hues on the hooded portion of the lid since they can highlight the hood.

Monolid Eyes: Use bright, shimmering colors to give the idea of depth and dimension. Avoid dark, matte colors, which can make the eyes appear smaller.

For round eyes, use darker tones on the outer corners and lighter shades on the inner corners to extend them. Avoid using too much shimmer, which can make the eyes appear rounder.

Almond eyes are suitable for most makeup looks. Experiment with various colors and techniques to improve your natural eye shape.

Applying Eyeliner for Various Looks

Winged Eyeliner: Begin by drawing a line along the upper lash line and extending it slightly beyond the outer corner of the eye. Make a wing by drawing a diagonal line from the outer corner back toward the eyelid, then fill in the space and connect it to the upper lash line.

Tightline: Use eyeliner along the upper waterline to make the lashes appear bigger and the eyes more defined.

Smudged or Smoky Eyeliner: Apply eyeliner to the upper and lower lash lines, then blend and soften with a smudge brush or your fingers to achieve a smoky appearance.

Tips to Volumize and Lengthen Lashes with Mascara

Apply a lash prep before mascara to increase length and volume.

Wiggle the Wand: To achieve maximum volume and length, wiggle the mascara wand from the base of the lashes all the way to the tips.

Layer Mascara: To add volume and length, apply numerous coats of mascara, allowing each to dry before applying the next.

Use a Lash Curler: Before using mascara, curl your lashes to lift and lengthen them.

Remove Excess Mascara: To minimize clumping, gently wipe any excess mascara from the wand before applying it.

Experiment with different eyeshadow colors, eyeliner styles, and mascara formulas to see what best suits your eye shape and intended look.

Choosing the proper lipstick and lip liner hues, applying lipstick evenly, preventing feathering, giving the illusion of bigger lips, and using long-lasting lip makeup procedures can all improve your entire makeup look. Here's a roadmap to help you accomplish these objectives:

Choosing Lipstick and Liner Shades

Skin Tone: Select lipstick tones that compliment your skin tone. Pinks and corals suit fair skin wonderfully. Rose or berry tints work well with medium complexion tones. For darker skin tones, choose rich browns and deep reds.

Lip Liner Matching: For a seamless effect, match your lip liner to the same hue as your lipstick. For a more versatile look, try a neutral lip liner that complements your natural lip color.

How to Apply Lipstick Evenly and Prevent Feathering

Exfoliate Lips: Before applying lipstick, exfoliate your lips to eliminate any dry or flaky skin.

Use a Lip Brush: To ensure uniform application, use a lip brush.

Blot and Layer: After applying the initial layer of lipstick, blot your lips with a tissue before adding a second coat for longer-lasting color.

Prevent Feathering: Before applying lipstick, outline your lips with a clear lip liner.

Creating the illusion of fuller lips

Overline Lips: Apply a lip liner slightly outside your natural lip line to give the appearance of bigger lips. For a more natural appearance, avoid overdoing it.

Use a Highlighter: Apply a little bit of highlighter to the center of your lips to make them appear larger.

Glossy Finish: Apply a lip gloss to the center of your lips to give volume and shine.

Long-lasting Lip Makeup Techniques

Select a long-lasting lipstick or lip stain for extended wear.

Set with Powder: After applying lipstick, softly dust translucent powder over your lips to seal the color.

Blot and Reapply: After applying lipstick, use a tissue to blot your lips before reapplying for longer-lasting color.

Use a Lip Primer: Apply a lip primer before lipstick to produce a smooth base and extend wear time.

Experiment with various lipstick and lip liner shades, application techniques, and finishes to see what best suits your style and preferences.

CHAPTER FOUR

Blending Techniques for a Smooth Makeup Application

Blend foundation, concealer, and other cream or liquid products with a damp makeup sponge or brush to get a smooth, airbrushed effect.

For eyeshadow, use a fluffy blending brush to blend colors together smoothly, focusing on the edges to avoid harsh lines.

To avoid streaks and hard lines, blend blush and bronzer gently along the cheekbones and temples.

Setting Makeup with Setting Spray to Create a Dewy Finish

To set your makeup, hold a setting spray about an arm's length away from your face and mist it all over. This extends the wear time of your makeup and provides a radiant finish.

Fixing Makeup Mistakes and Achieving a Perfect Look

Use a cotton swab or a small brush soaked in makeup remover to carefully erase any mistakes, such as smudged eyeliner or lipstick outside the lip line.

To get a perfect look, begin with a well-prepped base (clean, moisturized skin) and apply makeup in thin, even layers, increasing coverage as needed.

To achieve a smooth look, blend any harsh lines or uneven areas with a clean makeup sponge or brush.

Makeup Removal and Skincare Tips

To remove makeup, use a light makeup remover or cleaning oil, paying careful attention to the eye area and lips.

Finally, use a gentle cleanser to remove any residual makeup and pollutants.

After cleansing, moisturize your skin to keep it nourished and healthy.

Regular exfoliation helps to remove dead skin cells and maintain your skin smooth.

Use sunscreen every day to protect your skin from UV rays and premature aging.

Remember that practice makes perfect when it comes to makeup application. Experiment with various treatments and products to see what works best for you and your skin type.

Daytime Makeup for a Natural and Everyday Look

Begin with a hydrated face and use a light, tinted moisturizer or BB cream to create a natural-looking base.

Use concealer to mask any imperfections or dark circles.

Use a neutral makeup hue on your eyelids and mascara to define your lashes.

Apply a little of blush to the apples of your cheeks for a healthy flush.

For a more modest look, apply a sheer lip gloss or a neutral lipstick.

Evening Makeup For A More Dramatic Look

Start with a matte foundation to achieve a more finished look.

To enhance depth, apply a deeper eyeshadow hue to the crease and outer corners of your eyes.

Apply eyeliner to the top lash line and add false lashes for extra drama.

To achieve a sculpted look, contour your cheeks with bronzer.

For a standout finish, apply a bright lipstick or lip gloss.

Begin with a primer to guarantee that your makeup lasts throughout the occasion.

To get a flawless complexion, apply full-coverage foundation and concealer.

Apply a shimmering eyeshadow on your eyelids, then apply eyeliner and mascara for definition.

Contour and accentuate your features to achieve a sculpted effect.

Finish with a long-lasting lipstick or lip stain in a strong color that matches your clothing.

Tips for Long-Lasting Makeup and Touch-ups Throughout the Day

Use a beauty setting spray to seal in your makeup and make it last longer.

Carry pressed powder and blotting papers to touch up any oily areas during the day.

Maintain a compact makeup bag stocked with essentials such as lipstick, concealer, and mascara for quick touch-ups on the road.

Blot your lipstick with a tissue and reapply for a new look.

Avoid touching your face during the day to avoid smudging and smearing.

THE END

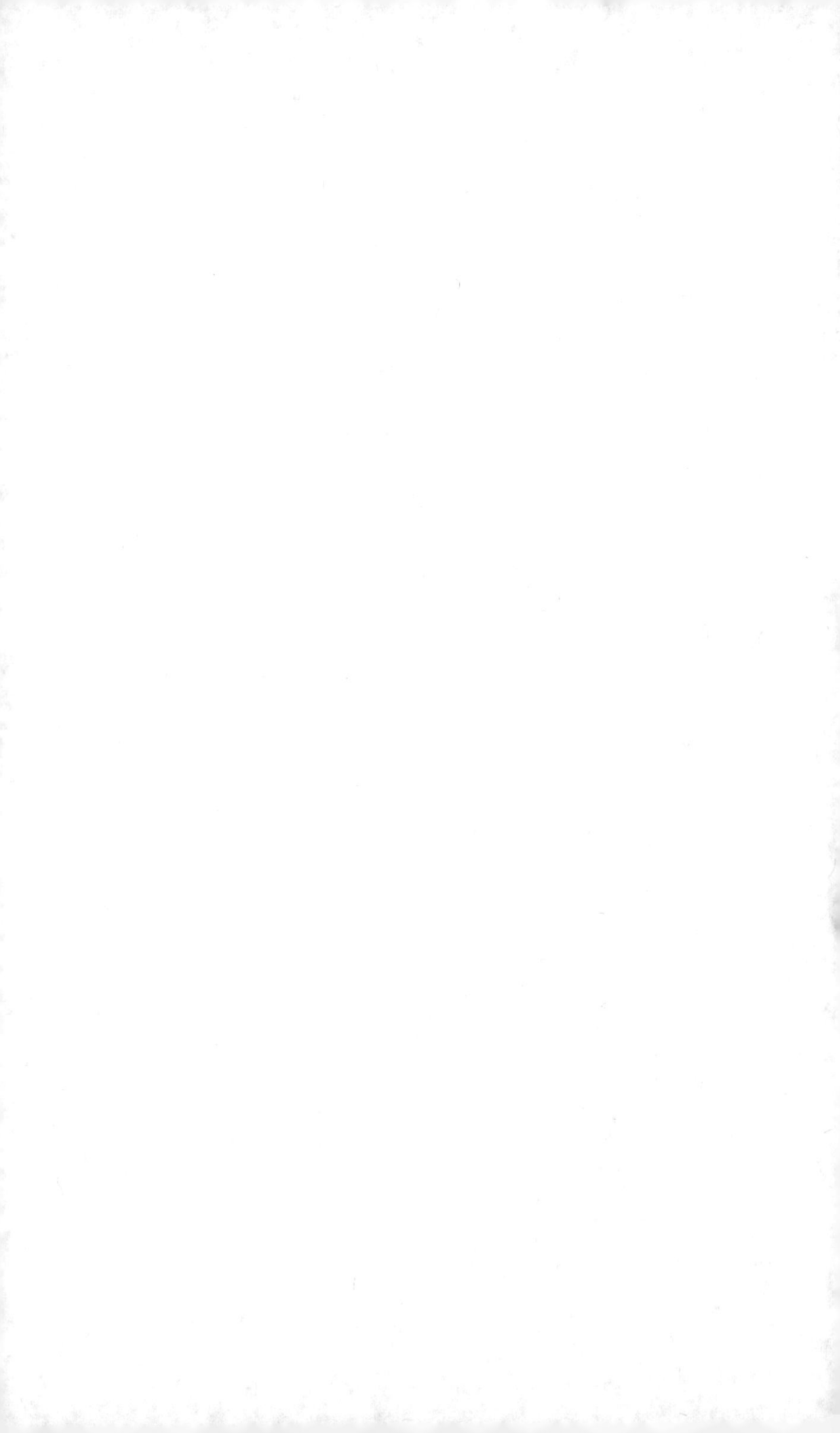

www.ingramcontent.com/pod-product-compliance
Lightning Source LLC
Chambersburg PA
CBHW061319250726
48653CB00002B/969